We Like to Grow Our Food

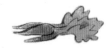

DENISE A. INCAO

Illustrations by Valentina Jaskina

The Family & World Health Series
KALINDI PRESS
Chino Valley, Arizona

Cover Image and Interior Illustrations: Valentina Jaskina: astound.us/publishing/artists/valentina-jaskina
Cover Design: Kubera Book Design, Prescott, Arizona
Interior Design and Layout: Kubera Book Design, Prescott, Arizona

ISBN: 978-1-935826-49-1

Kalindi Press
P.O. Box 4410
Chino Valley, AZ 86323
800-381-2700
http://www.kalindipress.com

This book was printed in China

For all the children of our
gracious Mother, Nature

For Parents, Teachers and Friends

A garden is a wonderful teacher, full of surprising and valuable gifts. *We Like to Grow Our Food* stresses the need for nurturance, patience and sharing—all vital life lessons for young children to hear about and for parents, teachers and friends to encourage. This book inspires us all to care for plants as living beings, just like the bugs and the animals that are also present in the garden. In simple words and with bright, playful illustrations, we learn how people, plants and animals are related and work together in the web of life. This early understanding gives our little ones a tremendous head start on their life journey.

In *We Like to Grow Our Food*, children hear about composting, the need for healthy soil, companion planting, beneficial insects and animals, and the joy of harvesting real, healthy food grown by little hands like theirs. Growing a food garden provides new opportunities for kids to learn about healthy choices and develop healthier eating habits. And, we all get to celebrate the essential bond with nature that is so easy to forget in a fast-food culture.

Growing your own food is not only fun and an adventure; it's good for the brain, the body, the soul and the Earth too. Children need to connect with soil, air, sunlight and the joys of nature that garden-making and food growing can provide. Get them started early, even if your garden is only a few pots on a backyard stairs or in a schoolyard.

Additional resources are listed at the end of this book for you to continue your learning and adventure.

The glory of gardening: hands in the dirt, head in the sun, heart with nature.
To nurture a garden is to feed not just the body, but the soul.

— **Alfred Austin** (English Poet, 1835 – 1913)

We like to grow our food. We can grow fresh veggies, fruits and herbs, with our own hands, and a little help.

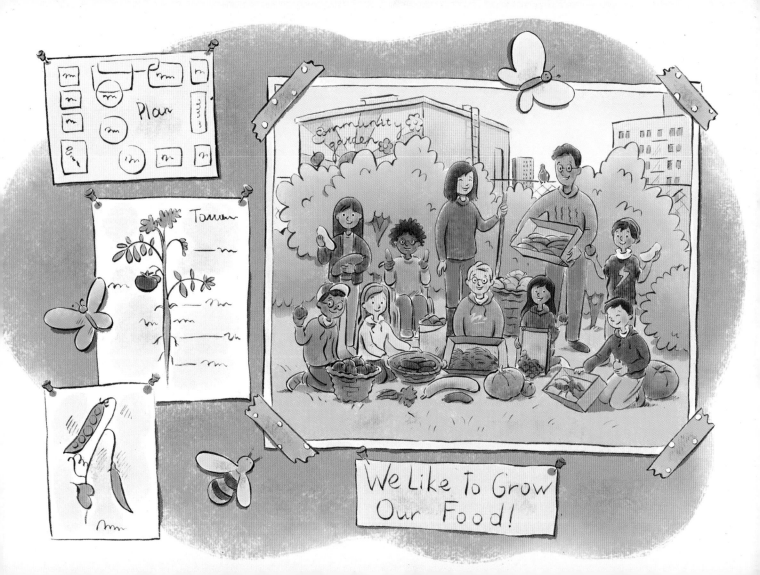

We plan our garden early. So grab those tools, buckets and boots! Dig up the soil and mix in organic compost – the nutritious food that young plants need.

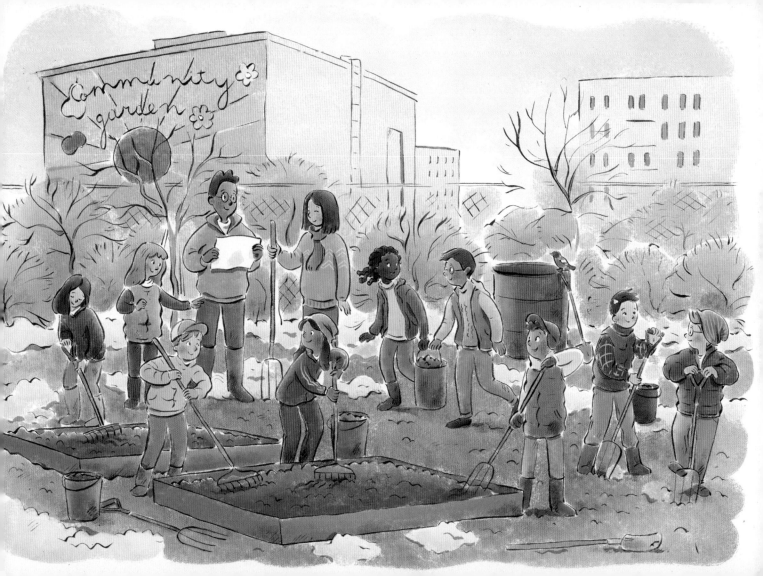

If springtime is warm enough, we can plant seeds right in the garden soil . . .

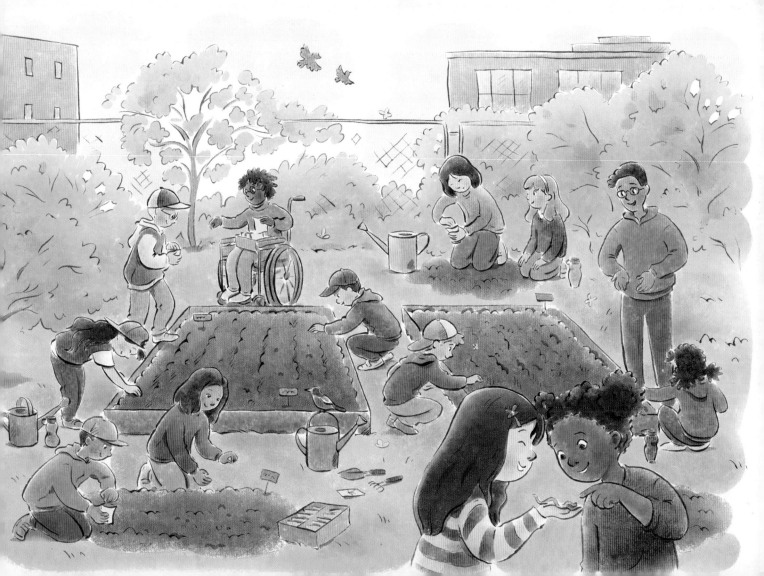

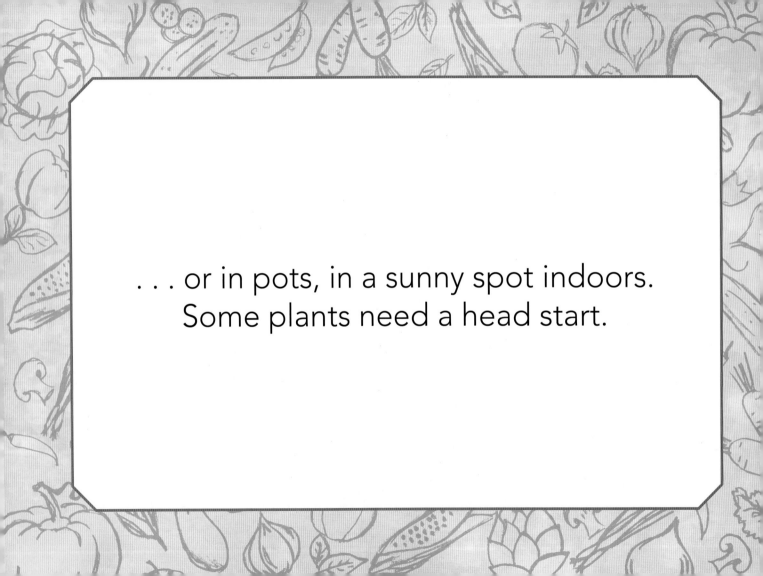

. . . or in pots, in a sunny spot indoors. Some plants need a head start.

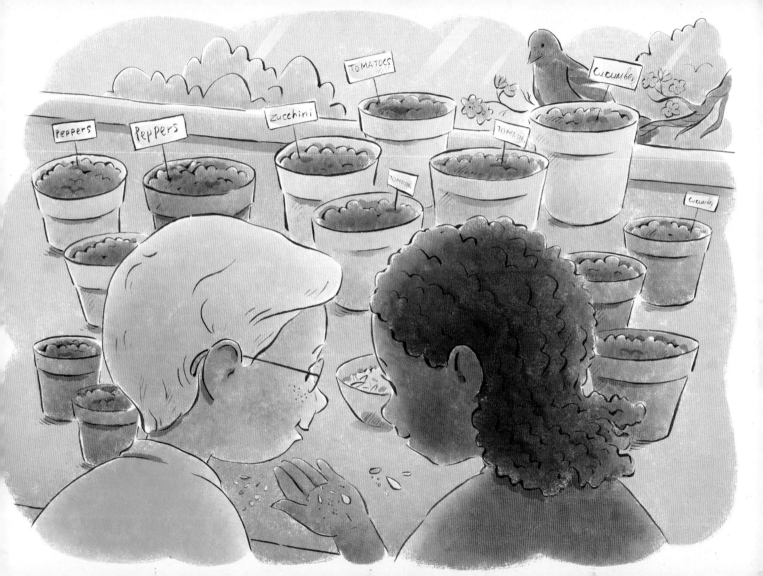

We water, we wait and we watch. Soon, when the time is just right, tiny sprouts pop into the daylight.

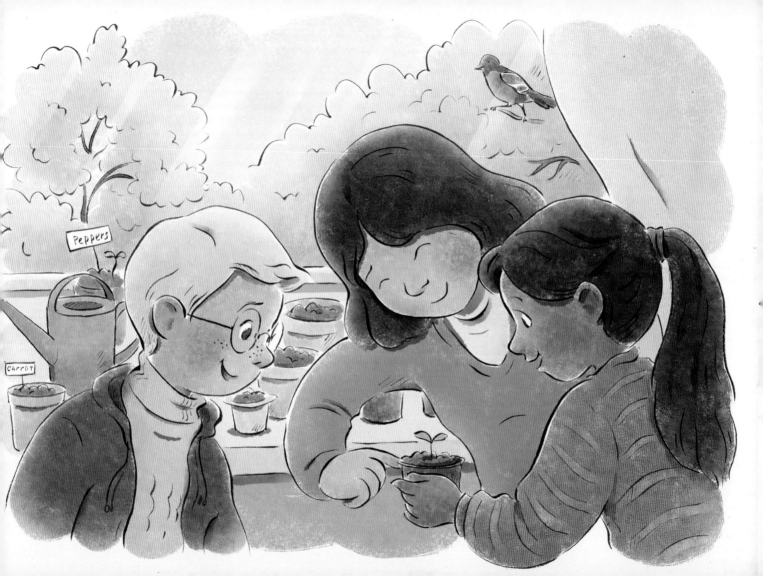

As seedlings grow, we make space around them for new roots, leaves and flowers. Baby plants grow quickly, just like children.

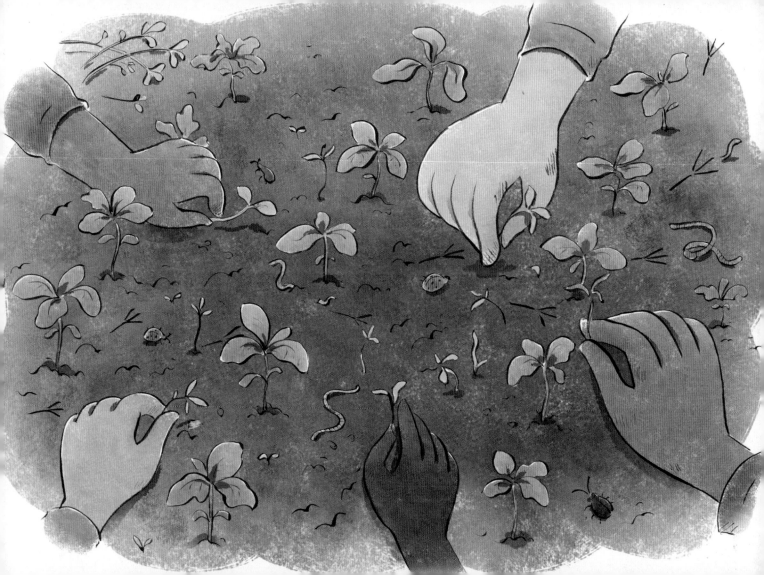

When the days are warmer and our little plants are bigger, out to the garden they go.

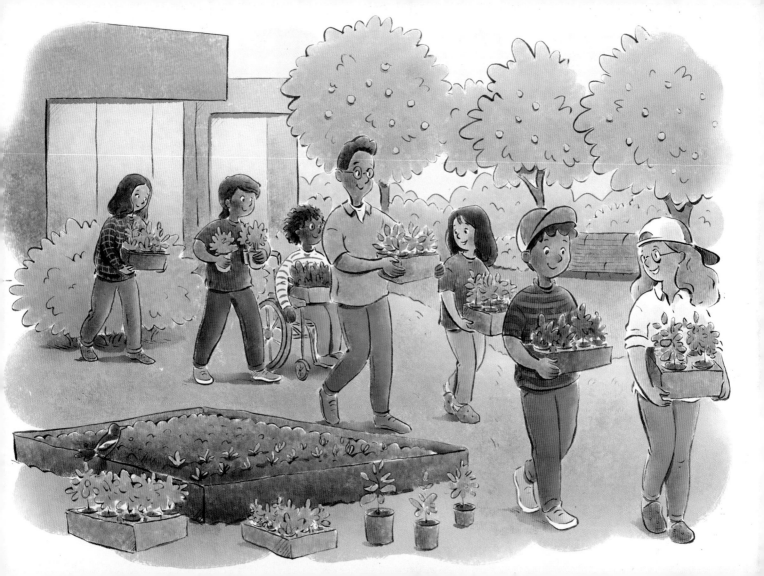

We plant tomatoes near carrots. Like us, plants have "besties" – good friends that share nutrients and protect them from pests.

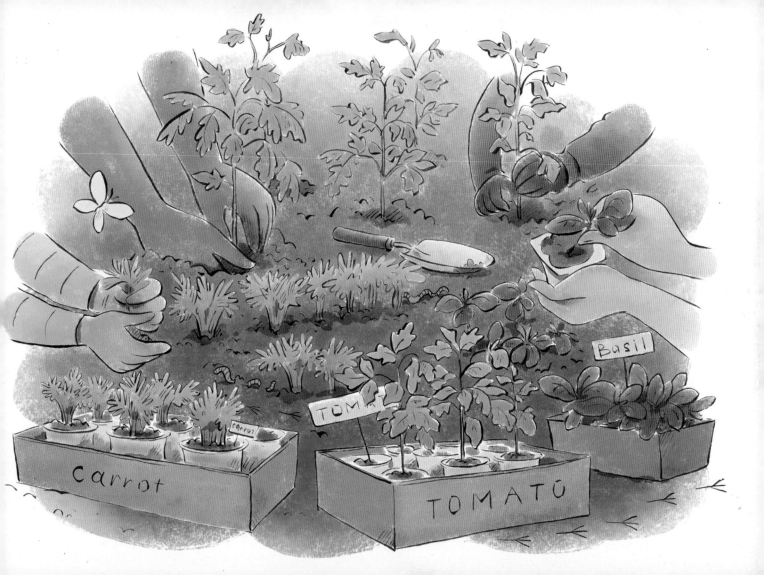

We care for and pay attention
to what our garden needs: weeding and
watering and feeding it with organic food.

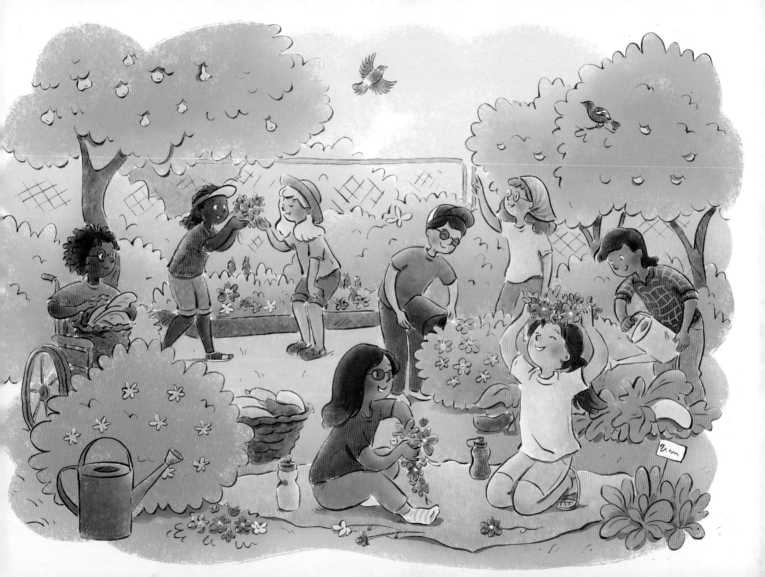

Some insects and animals help our garden plants too. They can help pollinate or keep hungry bugs from eating our food. Let's welcome them!

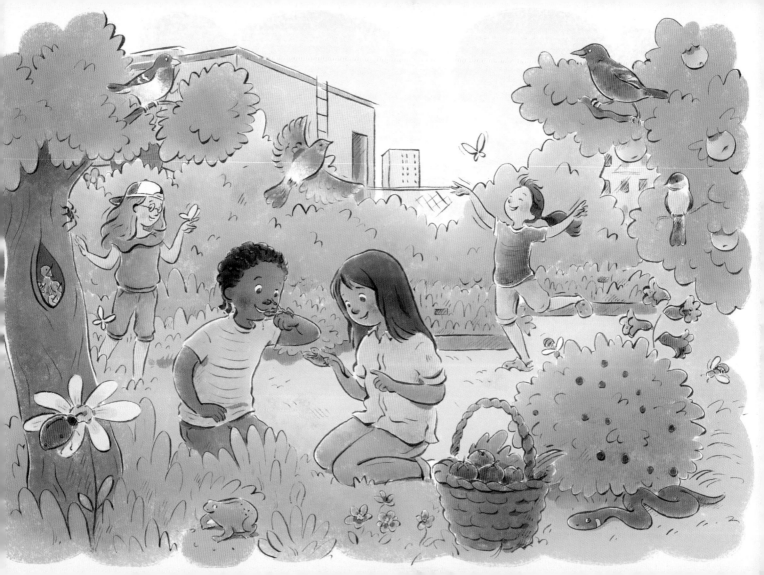

Harvesting is fun! We get yummy, nutritious food for our bodies, and good feelings from caring for nature.

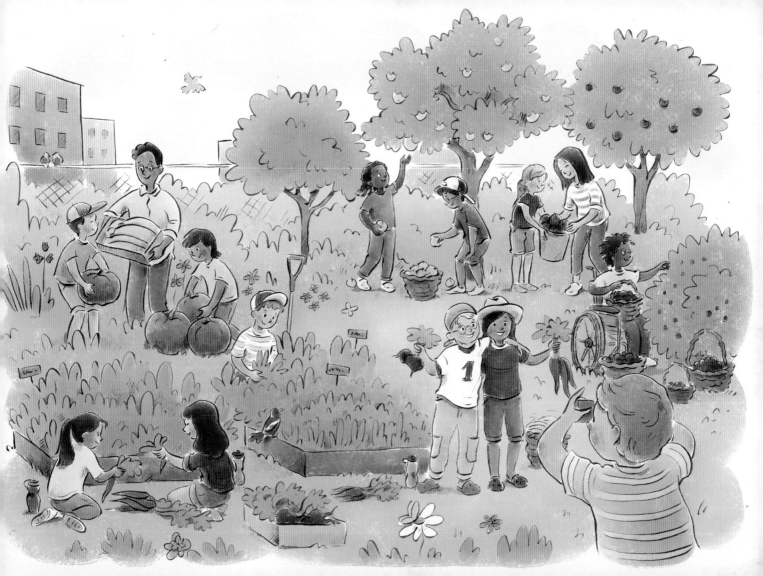

When the growing season's over,
we save some seeds to plant next spring,
and put our garden to bed for the winter.
We like to grow our food!

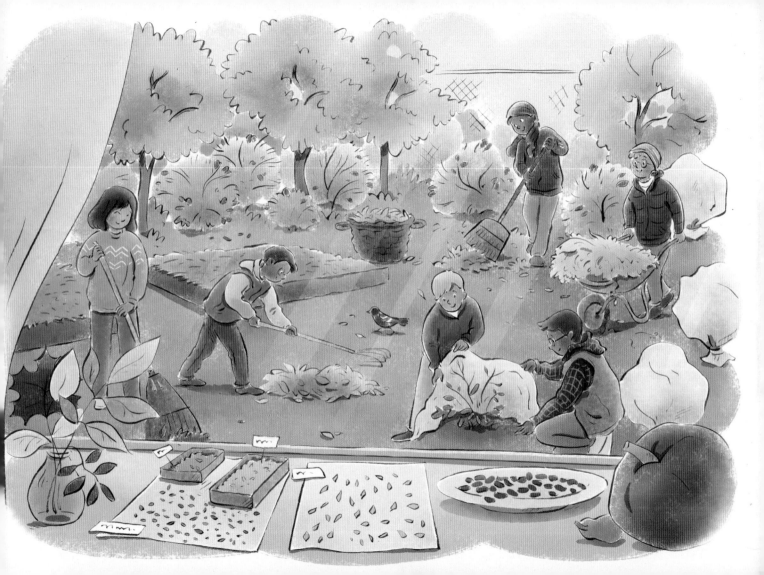

Resources for Parents, Teachers and Caregivers

Websites

https://www.wholekidsfoundation.org/
https://kidsgardening.org
https://www.fns.usda.gov/tn/team-nutrition-garden-resources

Books

Gardening with Kids:
Raskin, Ben. *Grow: A Family Guide to Growing Fruits and Vegetables*. Roost Books, 2017.

Companion Planting:
Carr, Anna. *Good Neighbors: Companion Planting for Gardeners*. Rodale Press, 1985.
Riotte, Louise. *Carrots Love Tomatoes: Secrets to Companion Planting for Successful Gardening*. Storey Publishing, 1998.

Beneficial Insects for Food Gardens:
Pfeffer, Wendy, and Steve Jenkins. *Wiggling Worms at Work*. HarperCollins, 2004.
Souza, D M. *Insects in the Garden*. Carolrhoda Books, 1991.
Starcher, Allison M. *Good Bugs for Your Garden*. Algonquin Books, 1998.

Pollination:
Kalman, Bobbie. *What Is Pollination?* Crabtree Publishing Company, 2010.
Heller, Ruth. *The Reason for a Flower: A Book About Flowers, Pollen, and Seeds (Explore!)*. Puffin Books:1999.

Composting:
Glaser, Linda and Shelley Rotner. *Garbage Helps Our Garden Grow: A Compost Story*. Millbrook Press, 2010.
Siddals, Mary M. K. and Ashley Wolff, *Compost Stew: An A to Z Recipe for the Earth*. Tricycle Press, 2010.

How Seeds Grow:
Fowler, Allan. *From Seed to Plant*. Children's Press (Scholastic), 2001.
Jordan, Helene J. *How a Seed Grows*. HarperCollins, 1992.

CONTACT INFORMATION

About the Author

Denise A. Incao holds a BFA in Sculptural Ceramics from Auburn University (Alabama), and a Master's degree in Expressive Ecopsychology from Prescott College (Arizona). She lives in northern Arizona with her husband and teenage daughter. Contact: www.deniseincao.com

About the Illustrator

Valentina Jaskina studied classical drawing, painting and graphic design at Novosibirsk Art College, in Siberia. Her work is often mixed technique: ink plus digital graphics. She lives in Novosibirsk, Siberia with her husband and two daughters.

About Kalindi Press

Kalindi Press, an affiliate of **Hohm Press**, proudly offers books in natural health and nutrition, as well as the acclaimed *Family Health* and *World Health Series* for children and parents, covering such themes as nutrition, dental health, reading, and environmental education.

Visit our website at: www.kalindipress.com
And: www.familyhealthseries.com